OIL OF OREGANO

Nature's Antiseptic
and Antioxidant

Barbara Schuetz

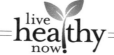

HEALTHY LIVING PUBLICATIONS
Summertown, Tennessee

Cover and interior design: Scattaregia Design

Healthy Living Publications,
a division of Book Publishing Company
PO Box 99
Summertown, TN 38483
888-260-8458
bookpubco.com

ISBN:978-1-57067-329-0

Printed in the United States of America

20 19 18 17 16   1 2 3 4 5 6 7 8 9

Library of Congress Cataloging-in-Publication Data

Names: Schuetz, Barbara, author.
Title: Oil of oregano : nature's antiseptic and antioxidant / Barbara Schuetz.
Description: Summertown, Tennessee : Healthy Living Publications, 2016. |
   Includes bibliographical references.
Identifiers: LCCN 2016013119 (print) | LCCN 2016014580 (ebook) | ISBN
   9781570673290 (pbk.) | ISBN 9781570678578 (E-book)
Subjects: LCSH: Essences and essential oils--Therapeutic use. |
   Oregano--Therapeutic use.
Classification: LCC RM666.A68 S38 2016 (print) | LCC RM666.A68 (ebook) | DDC
   615.3/4--dc23
LC record available at http://lccn.loc.gov/2016013119

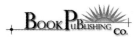

We chose to print this title on responsibly harvested paper stock certified by The Forest Stewardship Council, an independent auditor of responsible forestry practices. For more information, visit https://us.fsc.org.

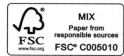

MIX
Paper from
responsible sources
FSC® C005010

CONTENTS

Introduction

As TV commercials rattle off the scary side effects of the latest drug on the market and the cost of health care causes some folks to turn to Grandma's home remedies, the world of herbal medicine is drawing a lot of interest, from brewing dried leaves for peppermint tea to inhaling the calming vapors of lavender essential oil. In 2012 the National Center for Health Statistics, part of the Centers for Disease Control and Prevention, found that over 33 percent of adults and about 12 percent of children in the United States had used alternative or complementary medicine in some form during the previous year. And those numbers have been growing. While herbal remedies are considered "alternative" medicine in North America, they're the norm in other parts of the world. According to the World Health Organization, 65 to 80 percent of people worldwide use herbal remedies as their primary form of health care.

Many herbal remedies have a long history, with some dating back to ancient times. But it wasn't until the early nineteenth century that scientists began studying the chemical compounds in plants. Today about one-fourth of all pharmaceutical drugs are derived from botanical sources. For instance, thymol, a beneficial extract obtained from the herb oregano, can be found in cough drops, topical cold remedies (such as VapoRub), and antiseptic mouthwash (such as Listerine). So it's not surprising that many health-conscious people are skipping the middleman (the over-the-counter product) and going directly to the source: oregano and the essential oil derived from it.

Although scientific research on oregano and other herbs is often limited to test tube studies, that hasn't stopped people from exploring the potential of botanical medicines. In 2013 alone, sales of herbal dietary supplements rose 8 percent, reaching $6 million, according to the American Botanical Council, which attributes the increase to our growing interest and confidence in the herbal market.

Concentrated essential oils distilled from herbs are readily available to consumers interested in aromatherapy, a term that applies to a range of holistic therapies that include inhalation, massage, and topical applications. Among the crop of popular options are lavender, peppermint, and tea tree essential oils. Oregano oil has also been amassing followers, as suppliers and health-related publications frequently tout it as a remedy for everything from colds and indigestion to fungal infections and arthritis pain. Even though oregano has been around for centuries, researchers are still learning about the potential benefits of its essential oil. The following pages explore what we know about oregano oil, what information is still speculative, and how this herbal remedy may be advantageous to our health.

Oregano: Joy of the Mountains

When most people hear the word oregano, pizza is usually the first image that comes to mind, so it's not surprising that the herb is often referred to as the "pizza spice." Its warm, spicy fragrance and pungent flavor have made it a staple in the kitchen, not only for pizza and other Italian favorites but also for vinaigrettes, stews, soups, and a variety of Mexican dishes. And because it's not difficult to grow, oregano is frequently a mainstay of both backyard and indoor window gardens.

But this herb is more than just a culinary essential. Oregano has traditionally been used worldwide as a remedy for digestive upset, inflammation, colds and flu, and respiratory problems, such as asthma and bronchitis. And Americans are catching on to that fact. Just Google "oregano" or "oregano oil" and you'll find an explosion of articles, blogs, and retailers espousing the benefits of what television's Dr. Oz has called "liquid gold."

Ancient Remedy

Oregano and its essential oil have long been referred to as "nature's antibiotic," the "prince of herbs," and even the "Mediterranean miracle" because of their seemingly endless list of potential benefits. Many of those benefits have been realized for ages and were recorded in the earliest natural histories by writers such as Pliny and Galen. Hippocrates, the ancient Greek physician who is considered the father of modern medicine, used oregano as an antiseptic and for treating digestive and respiratory conditions. Some sources credit him with naming the herb, which was also known as "wild marjoram" in earlier times. In some regions, oregano is still referred to as wild marjoram, while the actual herb marjoram is often referred to as "sweet marjoram."

Oregano may be associated with Italian food, but it probably originated in Greece and is native to the Mediterranean and Eurasia. The herb has been grown in Egypt for more than three thousand years and in England since the thirteenth century. Its name comes from the Greek words *oros*, meaning "mountain," and *ganos*, meaning "joy"—the joy of the mountains. Legend has it that the goddess Aphrodite created oregano as a symbol of happiness, and the herb was often included in ancient wedding ceremonies in which the bride and groom were crowned with laurels of oregano. It was also used as an aphrodisiac. Early Greeks used the leaves to make creams for treating sores and muscle aches and thought cows that grazed in fields of oregano produced more flavorful beef. They also believed that when wild marjoram (oregano) was combined with wild thyme and placed near milk pails, the herbs would keep the milk from going sour during thunderstorms.

Romans discovered oregano when they invaded Greece and have often been credited with introducing the herb to the rest of Europe. The eighteenth-century Irish herbalist John K'Eogh wrote of oregano's "hot, dry nature" and said it was good "against pains of the stomach and heart and also useful for coughs, pleurisy and obstructions of the lungs and womb, and it also comforts the head and nerves." The herb eventually found its way to China, where doctors have used it for centuries to relieve such conditions as diarrhea, fever, itchy skin, jaundice, nausea, and vomiting.

Oregano has been grown on American soil since colonial times, but it wasn't in widespread use until after World War II, when soldiers returned home raving about Italian food. Since then oregano use has continued to grow in popularity. It's estimated that Americans consume more than fourteen million pounds of oregano a year, and among herbs, it's one of the top imports in terms of both value and quantity.

Nutritional and Chemical Components

A member of the mint (*Lamiaceae* or *Labiatae*) family, oregano is related to both thyme and marjoram. Oregano boasts more than forty species, according to the Herb Society of America. Common oregano (*Origanum vulgare*) and marjoram (*Origanum majorana*) are often used interchangeably in cooking. However, their flavors have a subtle difference: oregano is peppery and zesty, while marjoram is sweeter and more delicate. Some producers of essential oil mistakenly use marjoram instead of oregano, but marjoram does not contain the key ingredient—carvacrol—that gives oregano oil its healing benefits (see page 9).

Oregano is a hardy perennial herb (an annual in colder climates) that can grow to about thirty inches tall and wide in the best conditions, although most reach eight to twelve inches in height. (See page 33 for planting and growing tips.) This fast-growing herb produces pretty white to purplish flowers. The entire plant—leaves, flowers, and stems—can be used for both culinary and medicinal purposes. The leaves are a rich source of vitamin K, which promotes bone growth, maintenance of bone density, and production of blood-clotting proteins. It's also a good source of dietary fiber, calcium, iron, manganese, vitamin E, and tryptophan, an essential amino acid.

Table 1. Vitamins in dried oregano (*Origanum vulgare*)

Vitamins	Per 100 grams	Per 1 teaspoon, ground
Folate	237 µg	4 µg
Niacin	4.640 mg	.084 mg
Riboflavin	0.528 mg	.010 mg
Thiamin	0.177 mg	.003 mg
Vitamin A	1701 IU	31 IU
Vitamin B-6	1.044 mg	.019 mg
Vitamin C	2.3 mg	0 mg
Vitamin E	18.26 mg	.33 mg
Vitamin K	621.7 µg	11.2 µg

Source: USDA National Nutrient Database for Standard Reference, accessed Sept. 4, 2015.

Table 2. Minerals in dried oregano (*Origanum vulgare*)

Minerals	Per 100 grams	Per 1 teaspoon, ground
Calcium	1,597 mg	29 mg
Iron	36.8 mg	.66 mg
Magnesium	270 mg	5 mg
Manganese	4.99 mg	.09 mg
Phosphorus	148 mg	3 mg
Potassium	1,260 mg	23 mg
Zinc	2.69 mg	.05 mg

Source: USDA National Nutrient Database for Standard Reference, accessed Sept. 4, 2015.

The chemical compounds found in oregano leaves' volatile, or essential, oil can vary, depending on the plant's geographic location and other factors. One study from France that analyzed the essential oil from leaves of the *Origanum compactum* species resulted in the identification of forty-six compounds, representing over 98 percent of the total composition. Carvacrol dominated at 36.46 percent, followed by thymol at 29.74 percent, and p-cymene at 24.31 percent. Carvacrol and thymol are phenols, which are a family of natural substances used in medicinal products. P-cymene is a monoterpene, a compound commonly found in aromatic herbs that enhances the therapeutic value of other components of the essential oil. Rosmarinic acid and beta-caryophyllene are also notable compounds found in *Origanums*. The oils of the various species can contain hundreds of additional chemical compounds, including pinene, limonene, linalool, and terpinene.

Carvacrol is responsible for much of oregano's medicinal prowess and thus has become one of the most extensively studied components of essential oils. This phenol is found in a number of plants, including thyme and wild bergamot, but it is most abundant in oregano—particularly *Origanum vulgare*. This chemical is known to inhibit the growth of bacteria and has been shown to reduce inflammation, protect DNA from damage, and prevent cancer cells from growing. Thanks to carvacrol's ability to kill germs, oregano has long been used to soothe gastrointestinal problems. Because the amount of carvacrol in oregano can vary widely, depending on such factors as growing conditions and the quality of the plant, it's difficult to say how much oregano or oregano oil can produce positive results. One thing is clear: more is *not* better. Too much carvacrol can be toxic.

Thymol is a naturally occurring compound with strong antimicrobial attributes when used alone or with carvacrol. It's known as an effective antiseptic, disinfectant, fungicide, and pesticide. Some mouthwashes and toothpastes contain thymol. It is also used to treat bronchitis. The late Norman R. Farnsworth, former director of the Program for Collaborative Research in the Pharmaceutical Sciences at the University of Illinois, Chicago, wrote that the active ingredients in thymol can help loosen phlegm in the lungs. Thymol can also help boost the immune system, shielding it against toxins; help prevent tissue damage; and encourage healing. In Germany, syrups that contain thymol are often prescribed for coughs. In the United States, thymol is used in cough drops as well as other over-the-counter remedies.

The Mint Family

The plant family *Lamiaceae*, or *Labiatae*, is made up of more than two hundred genera and more than seven thousand species. It is an important and popular group because of its herb plants, which are used for flavor, fragrance, and medicinal purposes. A few of the characteristics that most members of the mint family share are a strong aroma, tiny flowers, and volatile oils in their leaves and stems.

Historically, all mint-family herbs have been used for medicinal purposes. Horehound, for example, was once used to treat lung problems, and it's still included as an ingredient in cough drops and cough syrup. Like oregano, these herbs owe their medicinal attributes to volatile aromatic oils, such as camphor, carvacrol, limonene, and menthol, found in their leaves. In a German study, extracts of lemon balm, peppermint, and sage displayed strong activity against herpes simplex virus type 2 and also reduced the infectivity of HIV-1 viral particles, or virions. Research has shown that sage can help reverse heavy perspiration by 50 percent or more. And peppermint is an accepted cold remedy. Like oregano, thyme contains carvacrol; unlike oregano, marjoram does not contain phenols. Among other familiar herbs in this group are the following:

- basil
- bee balm
- catnip
- hyssop
- lavender
- mint
- rosemary
- savory

Benefits of Oregano Essential Oil

Essential oils have been used for centuries to treat a myriad of maladies, but only in recent years has their popularity as a natural remedy mushroomed in America. This has been primarily due to favorable scientific research along with consumers' penchant for natural ingredients in food, household products, and health care—despite the fact that essential oils are not regulated or approved by the US Food and Drug Administration. Even with only limited scientific research to rely on, many consumers swear by the effectiveness of essential oils.

Essential oils are extracted via steam distillation of the fresh herbs, particularly the flowers and leaves as well as other parts of the plant. It takes about one hundred pounds of oregano to make one pound of the essential oil. A wild Mediterranean variety of the species *Origanum vulgare* is generally considered to contain the highest amount of the oil's two key components, carvacrol and thymol, which provide oregano essential oil with its antibacterial, antifungal, anti-inflammatory, antioxidant, antiparasitic, and antiviral benefits. Inhaling oregano essential oil's intense, camphor-like scent is said to help balance a person's energy, but because the aroma is pungent and strong, it's recommended for only short-term use. Oregano essential oil is growing in popularity as a topical remedy, and although some sources also suggest ingesting a diluted version of the oil, most experts strongly advise against this and recommend using it only externally because of its toxicity. Below are some of the conditions that oregano essential oil is purported to help. Keep in mind that there is no empirical evidence yet to substantiate the efficacy of oregano essential oil for most of these conditions. However, there is a growing body of research that has reported positive results for the oil's capacity as an effective natural-healing agent. In addition, several studies have demonstrated the oil's potential as an antibacterial, antifungal, anti-inflammatory, antioxidant, antiparasitic, and antiviral.

• acne	• bronchitis	• earache
• allergies	• canker sores	• eczema
• arthritis	• colds and flu	• fatigue
• asthma	• cold sores	• gastritis
• athlete's foot	• congestion	• gum disease
• bloating	• dandruff	• hay fever
• boils	• diarrhea	• headache/migraine

- heartburn
- insect bites and stings
- menstrual cramps
- muscle/joint pain
- negative effects of menopause
- oily skin
- poison ivy
- psoriasis
- rhinitis
- ringworm
- rosacea
- sinusitis
- sore throat
- sprains
- toenail fungus
- toothache
- upset stomach
- urinary tract infection
- varicose veins
- warts and skin tags
- yeast infection (candida)

Antibacterial

Several studies have confirmed oregano oil's ability to kill a variety of bacteria, and scientists continue to explore its potential in this area. For example, oregano essential oil has shown promise in preventing food-borne illnesses caused by such pathogens as *E. coli*, *Listeria*, *Salmonella*, and *Shigella dysenteriae*. Adding oregano to foods may not only help kill bacteria but may also alleviate food-poisoning symptoms.

With more research, oregano oil and other medicinal herbs could be the go-to remedies for fighting infections as more and more strains of bacteria become resistant to antibiotics. A number of germs are already showing resistance to vancomycin, an antibiotic used to treat *Clostridium difficile* and other life-threatening bacterial infections among hospital patients. Vancomycin is considered the most potent antibiotic available and is typically only used as a last resort. In *The Atlantic*, Cyril Gay, a highly regarded researcher, veterinarian, and microbiologist with the US Department of Agriculture's Agricultural Research Services, stated, "The loss of antibiotics due to antimicrobial resistance is potentially one of the most important challenges the medical and animal health communities will face in the twenty-first century." The advantage of nature-based remedies like oregano oil is that bacteria do not develop a resistance to them (see box, page 14).

In a 2008 study conducted in China, researchers determined that the phenols carvacrol and thymol significantly inhibited the growth of *E. coli* cells by permeating the cell membrane, which ultimately led to the loss of membrane potential. And a team of researchers in Portugal found that *Origanum vulgare* was effective against forty-one strains of *Listeria monocytogenes*, a bacterium found in contaminated food. *Listeria* can cause a serious infection that primarily affects older adults, pregnant women, newborns, and adults with weakened immune systems. It's an important public health issue in the United States, but the risk can be reduced with the use of safe food preparation, consumption, and storage.

British and Indian scientists tested the essential oil of Himalayan oregano and found its antibacterial properties can even kill methicillin-resistant *Staphylococcus aureus* (MRSA). Known as a superbug, MRSA is more difficult to treat than most staph infections because it is resistant to common antibiotics. The scientists were aware that Mediterranean oregano oil was a powerful antimicrobial, but no one had tested this variety of oregano oil, which is common *Origanum vulgare* that grows in the mountains. The results of the testing showed that the oregano oil was more effective at killing MRSA than eighteen antibiotics.

At Georgetown University, two studies pitted oregano oil—and particularly the ingredient carvacrol—against three traditional antibiotics: streptomycin, penicillin, and vancomycin. The results showed that the oil could reduce bacterial infections as effectively as the antibiotics. Researcher Harry Preuss combined the oil with *Staphylococcus* bacteria, and the oregano oil, at low doses, inhibited the growth of the bacteria as effectively as the three pharmaceutical drugs. In the second study, eighteen mice were infected with the staph bacteria. Six of the mice received the oil for a month, and three of them survived. Six received carvacrol diluted in olive oil and only survived twenty-one days. (The other six received only olive oil, and one survived.) This demonstrated that there are other compounds besides carvacrol in oregano oil that have antibacterial properties.

Beating Drug-Resistant Bacteria

According to the US Food and Drug Administration, almost all of the major bacterial infections in the world are becoming resistant to antibiotics. The World Health Organization calls this rise in drug-resistant bacteria one of the world's most serious health crises. In fact, in September 2014, US president Barack Obama's administration announced a set of federal actions to combat the rise of antibiotic-resistant bacteria, citing the following statistics from the Centers for Disease Control and Prevention:

- Antibiotic-resistant infections are associated with twenty-three thousand deaths and two million illnesses in the United States each year.
- The impact of antibiotic-resistant infections on the national economy includes up to $35 billion in lost productivity due to sick days and hospitalization.

In March 2015, the administration released the comprehensive plan, which aims to enhance diagnosis and treatment in order to limit the spread of these bacteria.

Experts point to the overuse of antibiotics as the reason for this rise in so-called superbugs. Many of the antibiotics prescribed to people and to animals are unnecessary, the National Institutes of Health explains. Antibiotics work against bacterial infections but not viruses. So when we take an antibiotic for a viral infection, the drug won't affect the virus but instead will destroy bacteria in the body. The bacteria that survive grow and spread, even to other people. Over time the bacteria continue to thrive and the pharmaceuticals become less effective.

As today's antibiotics continue to lose their efficacy, scientists have undertaken additional research on herbs and their essential oils, hoping that these natural remedies can provide a potential solution to this global problem. Why herbs? Because of their highly complex chemical structure, oregano and other medicinal herbs are naturally equipped to combat bacteria and make it more difficult for the bacteria to fight back. In a 2014 interview, herbalist Stephen Harrod Buhner, author of *Herbal Antibiotics: Natural Alternatives for Treating Drug-Resistant Bacteria,* explained it this way: "With a pharmaceutical, the bacteria analyze [its] single compound and generate solutions to it, which they then pass on to other bacteria. Plants, on the other hand, generate multiple compounds that deactivate resistance mechanisms in the bacteria and enhance the activity of the plant's natural antibacterials. Bacteria cannot easily counteract that kind of complexity."

While several studies, including those mentioned in this chapter, have explored the feasibility of using essential oils instead of antibiotics, an article in *Open Microbiology Journal* proposed the idea of using antibiotics and essential oils in combination. Author and researcher Polly Soo Xi Yap writes that combining conventional antimicrobial agents with essential oils sometimes surpasses the essential oil's individual performance, producing enhanced antimicrobial activity. The combined use also reduces the minimum effective dose of the antibiotic in treating infections, which in turn decreases the possibility of adverse side effects from the antibiotic. Although studies provide only limited evidence of essential oils' resistance to bacteria, Yap adds, "It is likely that the multi-component nature of essential oils may reduce the potential of the occurrence of essential oils resistance because numerous targets need to adapt to hamper the effects of the essential oils." While more research is needed, Yap concludes, "There are plenty of possibilities for the essential oils to be used in combination with antibiotics as new treatment modalities to the bacterial infections."

Antifungal

Several in vivo (human) and in vitro (test tube) studies have shown that oregano oil—and its ingredient thymol—can stand up to a range of fungi, including *Candida albicans*, which causes candida, a fungal infection. In a 1999 study, two university researchers in Santa Fe, Argentina, tested basil, coriander, mint, oregano, and sage essential oils for their inhibitory effects on yeast and fungi growth by incubating cultures in a broth of yeast extract and sucrose. Oregano essential oil proved to be the strongest, completely inhibiting fungal growth.

A team of university researchers in Brazil studied the in vitro activity of oregano (*Origanum vulgare*) oil against sixteen *Candida* species. The test tube samples, from female dogs and a capuchin monkey, all proved sensitive to the essential oil. The scientists concluded that the antifungal activity of oregano essential oil against the *Candida* species suggests that it may represent an alternative treatment for the condition.

In a 2011 study, Spanish researchers found that surface application of oregano oil on fermented, dry-cured sausages reduced mold contamination without significantly affecting the drying process. The oil also helped improve the meat's texture.

Anti-inflammatory

Inflammation is the body's response to injury or infection. Chronic inflammation is associated with increased episodes of heart attacks and autoimmune disorders, such as diabetes, lupus, multiple sclerosis, and rheumatoid arthritis. Oregano oil is rich in rosmarinic acid, a polyphenol that's known to have anti-inflammatory action. The acid has been shown to decrease the number of neutrophils and eosinophils, two types of white blood cells that in increased numbers can cause inflammation associated with asthma and allergies. Historically, oregano oil has been used as a remedy for such inflammatory conditions as asthma, croup, and rheumatoid arthritis.

A Japanese clinical trial studied patients with seasonal allergic rhino-conjunctivitis who were given daily doses for twenty-one days of either 200 milligrams of rosmarinic acid, 50 milligrams of rosmarinic acid, or a placebo. Compared to the placebo, the rosmarinic acid delivered significant decreases in symptoms for patients who recorded their symptoms daily.

In 2009 scientists at Bonn University in Germany and Eidgenössische Technische Hochschule in Zurich, Switzerland, identified another active ingredient in oregano that can ease inflammation: beta-caryophyllene (E-BCP). Although E-BCP is found naturally in many spices and food plants, its benefit to humans had not yet been studied. In this trial, Swiss researchers injected E-BCP into the inflamed paws of ten mice. The ingredient helped seven of the ten mice, or 70 percent, recover from the inflammation. The study, published in the United States in the *Proceedings of the National Academy of Sciences*, also showed that E-BCP could be effective in deterring bone degeneration associated with osteoporosis.

In yet another study, researchers found that oregano extracts and constituents can suppress inflammation both in a test tube and in animals. Thymol inhibited the release of the pancreatic enzyme elastase, which is a sign of inflammatory disease activity, from human immune cells. Scientists concluded that the anti-inflammatory and antioxidant characteristics of thymol can be beneficial in controlling the inflammatory processes present in many types of infections.

Antioxidant

It's generally accepted that oregano oil contains very high concentrations of antioxidants, which help protect cells against the effects of free radicals and improve the ability to fight infection. Free radicals are unstable oxygen molecules that steal electrons from other molecules, and they are a factor in degenerative conditions, such as arthritis, cancer, and heart disease. They may also be involved in the aging process. Howard Greenspan, an AIDS researcher, notes that increasing antioxidant intake can help maintain immune function in people who are HIV-positive. Drinking abundant amounts of antioxidant tea, including tea made from oregano (see recipe, page 36), can help achieve that goal. Research has shown that the antioxidant activity of oregano and other plants in the mint family is due in part to rosmarinic acid, which also has antiviral and anti-inflammatory properties (see Anti-inflammatory, page 16).

For a study at the University of Split in Croatia, researchers from the school's Department of Biochemistry and Food Chemistry examined the antioxidant properties of oregano oil in relation to its chemical composition using three different methods. The tests confirmed that oregano essential oil has remarkable antioxidant properties. The scientists found that carvacrol and thymol are responsible for the antioxidant effect, but they also felt that there was a possible synergistic effect among the oxygen-containing compounds. These findings show that oregano oil could be a potential resource of natural antioxidants in the food industry.

Just how remarkable is oregano as an antioxidant? According to a 2001 herbal study by the Agricultural Research Service (ARS), the chief research agency of the US Department of Agriculture, three types of oregano—Greek, Italian, and Mexican—scored highest in antioxidant activity, attributable to their high levels of the ingredient rosmarinic acid. "Their activity was stronger than that of vitamin E and comparable to the food preservative BHA against fat oxidation," writes Rosalie Marion Bliss for ARS. Two researchers tested twenty-seven culinary herbs and twelve medicinal herbs. The test, called oxygen radical absorbance capacity, or ORAC (see box, page 19), measured the ability of the herb to disarm oxidizing compounds, a by-product of metabolism in our bodies. Other herbs, such as dill and winter savory, were only one-half to one-third as potent in antioxidant activity.

James Duke, a botanist who specializes in medicinal plants and the author of *The Green Pharmacy*, conducted his own investigation of sixty members of the mint family. He found that wild oregano was among the richest in antioxidant properties.

Oregano's antioxidant compounds have also shown promise in their ability to protect against oxidation of low-density lipoproteins (LDL, or "bad" cholesterol), which is a key factor in heart disease. A 2007 study tested both the essential oils and tea infusions of oregano (*Origanum vulgare*), thyme (*Thymus vulgaris*), and wild thyme (*Thymus serpyllum*). The protective effect of the oils is due to the presence of thymol and carvacrol, and in the tea infusions, the protective effect is the consequence of large amounts of polyphenols, including rosmarinic acid, and flavonoids, such as quercetin and luteolin. The findings, according to researchers, may have positive implications for the effect of these compounds on lowering LDL.

Tempering these encouraging outcomes is a clinical trial from 2006 in which scientists at the University of Helsinki in Finland investigated the antioxidant effects of oregano oil in healthy, nonsmoking men. Every day for four weeks the volunteers consumed mango-orange juice (a placebo), mango-orange juice enriched with 300 milligrams of phenolic compounds from oregano extract, or mango-orange juice enriched with 600 milligrams of the compounds from oregano extract. Researchers noted a marked increase in the excretion of phenolic compounds in the 600-milligram group; however, there were no effects on the biomarkers of lipid peroxidation. So although there were high amounts of oregano extract in the body, free radicals were still dominant.

Is ORAC a Viable Measurement?

Some herbal literature points to oregano oil's oxygen radical absorption capacity (ORAC) as being four times greater than blueberries and as much as twelve times greater than other produce. The ORAC of a food or supplement is determined by a lab test that, in simple terms, involves placing a sample of the food in a test tube with molecules that generate free radical activity—a sort of good guy/bad guy showdown. Scientists measure how well the sample's collective antibiotics protect the molecules from the free radicals and come up with the "total antioxidant capacity." The less free radical damage there is, the higher the food's ORAC.

Table 3. ORAC values for a sampling of foods

Items ranked on the basis of 100 grams	µmol TE/100g (micromol Trolox Equivalent per 100 grams)
Oregano, dried	200,129
Açai berries, freeze-dried	102,700
Cocoa powder, unsweetened	80,933
Sorghum bran, red	71,000
Goji berries	25,300
Oregano, fresh	13,978
Blueberries	6,552

Source: modernsurvivalblog.com.

In November 2007, the USDA reported ORAC values for 277 food items, and in May 2010 it added another forty-nine food items to its database. The values quickly became a tool for health-conscious consumers as well as marketers. Two years later, however, the USDA pulled the plug and removed the database from its website "due to mounting evidence that the values indicating antioxidant capacity have no relevance to the effects of specific bioactive compounds, including polyphenols, on human health." The press release further noted that the ORAC numbers were "routinely misused by food and dietary supplement manufacturing companies to promote their products and by consumers to guide their food and dietary supple-ment choices." In addition, ORAC testing methods were found to be inconsistent. In its closing paragraph, the USDA stated, "There is no evidence that the beneficial effects of polyphenol-rich foods can be attributed to the antioxidant properties of these foods."

Ray Sahelian, medical doctor and author of *Mind Boosters*, explained that marketers could exaggerate the numbers when promoting their products. By putting the ORAC value on the product label, food manufacturers would imply that the food has a high antioxidant capacity, but he cautioned that the measurements do not necessarily predict how a food will react in our bodies. Therefore, Sahelian advised consumers not to base their decisions about which foods or supplements to use solely on ORAC values.

Ronald Prior, a research chemist and adjunct professor at the University of Arkansas, who worked on the ORAC study, responded to the USDA's removal of the database: "It is unfortunate but true that numbers obtained from ORAC analysis have sometimes been misused, but that does not necessarily mean that the information is not useful if used appropriately." He went on to say that "statements to the effect that 'There is no evidence that the beneficial effects of polyphenol-rich foods can be attributed to the antioxidant properties of these foods' are not consistent with the scientific evidence." Prior then cited a study published in *Cancer Causes Control* (2012) that concluded: "Using the ORAC database, after adjusting for major covariates, we found decreased risks for the highest tertile of total phenolic intake compared with the lowest . . . suggesting that total phenolic consumption may decrease endometrial cancer risk."

Antiparasitic

In one of the few human trials involving oregano oil, thirty-three adults with chronic gastrointestinal issues were tested for parasites, and enteric parasites (*Blastocystis hominis*, *Entamoeba hartmanni*, and *Endolimax nana*) were found in fourteen of the patients. Those with parasites were administered four drops of emulsified Mediterranean oregano oil three times a day (a total of 600 milligrams) at meals. After six weeks, the *Entamoeba hartmanni* (four cases), *Endolimax nana* (one case), and *Blastocystis hominis* (eight cases) had completely disappeared.

Antiviral

As an antiviral, oil of oregano has exhibited the potential to fight tough, extremely difficult-to-control viruses. Researchers at the University of Arizona found that oregano oil and carvacrol can help kill the human norovirus, the leading cause of acute gastroenteritis, responsible for more than 267 million outbreaks worldwide each year, including 21 million in the United States. Norovirus is highly contagious and quickly spreads in closed places, such as cruise ships, schools, nursing homes, hospitals, and restaurants. It is transmitted via person-to-person contact as well as through contaminated food and water. Norovirus poses a serious health threat, especially to children, the elderly, and people with compromised immune systems or other medical issues. Side-by-side experiments involving oregano oil and carvacrol produced statistically significant reductions in the virus numbers within fifteen minutes of exposure. With increased time exposure, however, the carvacrol was far more effective—99.99 percent effective, in fact.

These findings exhibit carvacrol's potential as a natural food-and-surface sanitizer to control human norovirus by inactivating the pathogens before they enter the body. Researchers envision using carvacrol as a sanitizer because, unlike products such as bleach, it could be used on foods and kitchen surfaces without doing harm to humans. Although it doesn't act as quickly as bleach, carvacrol leaves a longer-lasting, protective residue on surfaces.

Other Research

In a paper on the potential health benefits of oregano oil, Keith W. Singletary, professor emeritus of nutrition at the University of Illinois, Urbana, says it's clear that oregano's chemical compounds can suppress the growth of a wide range of microorganisms in vitro. There is also evidence that its bioactive components may suppress inflammation and improve blood glucose and lipid regulation. But these are still "potentials" since human trials are generally lacking. Most researchers do agree, however, that the results of their studies warrant additional testing and that oregano and its essential oil show promise as a remedy for a variety of conditions.

Some herbalists and medical professionals already sing the praises of oregano oil. Clinical herbalist Michelle Lynde says it's the "gold standard of natural medicine." Cass Ingram, author of *The Cure Is in the Cupboard: How to Use Oregano for Better Health*, has called oil of oregano the "Rolls Royce of natural antiseptics." Some practitioners have even referred to it as the "magic healing oil."

Oregano oil got an additional nod when Mehmet Oz, a New York cardiothoracic surgeon, featured it in a segment of *Dr. Oz*, his popular daytime TV show. He called the oil "liquid gold," pointing to its antibiotic properties and its ability to kill bacteria and stave off viruses, fungi, and parasites.

Following are some further ways that oregano oil has shown potential:

Appetite control. Oregano's use as an appetite suppressant and stimulant dates back to ancient times. A 1997 study showed that when .27 percent oregano was added to pasta sauce, study participants increased the amount of food they ate. Raising the amount to .56 percent, however, had the opposite effect, and their food consumption decreased.

Cancer. A test tube trial at the University of Central Florida found that several components of oregano, including aristolochic acid I and II, could possibly have an effect against leukemia and other types of cancer.

Another study showed that oregano extracts were able to protect cells from oxidative stress damage and radiation-induced DNA damage. Thymol has shown that it can suppress melanoma cells in a test tube. But much more research is necessary to confirm that oregano oil has potential anti-cancer benefits.

Diabetes. With type 2 diabetes affecting so many Americans, a team at the University of Illinois, Urbana-Champaign, undertook a study to find out whether herbs can offer a natural way to help lower blood glucose as an alternative to high-priced prescription drugs. The researchers tested extracts from both commercial and greenhouse-grown rosemary, marjoram, and Greek and Mexican oregano for their ability to inhibit enzymes that play a role in insulin secretion or insulin signaling. The greenhouse herbs contained more polyphenols and flavonoids than the commercial extracts. Greenhouse-grown rosemary, marjoram, and Mexican oregano proved to be the best inhibitors of the insulin-secretion enzyme, while commercial rosemary, marjoram, and Mexican oregano were better inhibitors of the insulin-signaling enzyme. Human studies are now needed to better understand the role of these herbs in diabetes prevention.

Farming. Oil of oregano is proving to be a boon for some farmers as well. According to a *New York Times* story, a Pennsylvania farmer swears by oregano oil to fight off bacterial infections in his chickens, without resorting to antibiotics. Scott Sechler feeds his flock a special diet laced with oregano oil and a touch of cinnamon. He uses a brand of oregano oil produced by Ropapharm International, a Dutch firm, and Sechler stated that nothing he has tried has worked as well as the oil.

In 1999 the German pharmaceutical company Bayer conducted trials on an oregano oil product called Ropadiar, and it outperformed four of Bayer's products in controlling diarrhea in piglets caused by *E. coli*. According to a Bayer physician, the oregano oil was more effective and provided quicker results, and the animals looked healthier too.

Food preservative. Because of oregano's antibacterial properties, scientists have looked into the possibility of using the herb as a natural food preservative. A team of researchers in Israel treated a whole Asian sea bass with the essential oils of oregano (*Origanum vulgare*) and thyme (*Thymus vulgaris*). The oils successfully inhibited any bacterial growth and prevented spoilage, extending the shelf life of the bass in cold storage to thirty-three days.

Natural Food Additive

Food-borne illnesses have become a worldwide public health problem. Each year more than thirty species of pathogens result in more than nine million cases of food-borne illness. To control this growing problem, manufacturers rely on synthetic food additives to extend the shelf life of their products. Because of the generally negative opinion consumers have about such additives, manufacturers are looking for natural alternatives. The antibacterial properties of oregano and other essential oils make them a choice worth considering. In Europe, a number of compounds, including carvacrol and thymol, have already been approved as registered "flavorings."

Although studies have shown the antibacterial potential of oregano oil and other oils, such as cilantro, their use has been limited because "high concentrations are needed to achieve sufficient antimicrobial activity," according to an article in *Frontiers in Microbiology*. The components in essential oils have also been hampered by interactions with the starch, fat, and proteins in food.

Using Oregano Oil

There is a plethora of suggested uses for oil of oregano; however, keep in mind that most are not scientifically proven. Still, many herbalists, health care providers, and consumers have found the oil a safe and effective solution for certain maladies and a beneficial alternative to pharmaceuticals. As with any remedy, natural or chemical, be sure to review the safety information on page 31 and talk to your health care professional before using the oil, particularly if you have diabetes, high blood pressure, or any other condition for which you are being treated.

Buying the Oil

Oregano oil's long list of potential benefits make it a great all-around supplement to have in your "medicine" cabinet. Of course, quality is of utmost importance, so always read the labels before purchasing.

Shopping online will give you a number of choices, and by using Google or Amazon, you'll be able to compare each brand's attributes and prices. Shopping at a retail store will give you the opportunity to smell the oil and possibly talk to someone who has used the products.

Some retailers offer oil infusions rather than essential oils, and there's a big difference between the two. Essential oils are steam distilled from raw plants, which release vapors that eventually condense into the liquid concentrate. These concentrated oils must be diluted before using. Infusions, which are much less potent than the essential oils, are produced by placing raw or dried leaves in a container of olive or another type of oil and allowing the plant's properties to steep into the oil. Infusions do not need to be diluted. You can even make an infusion at home (see page 41).

Below are some tips to help you wade through the number of brands in stores and online.

Carvacrol's the key. The percentage of carvacrol can range from 30 percent to over 80 percent. Solutions with higher percentages of the ingredient generally cost more but are more effective.

Check the species. *Origanum vulgare*, which grows wild in the Himalayas and the mountains of Greece and Turkey, is generally considered the species with the most therapeutic properties, but some oils are derived from other varieties. Comparable varieties include *Origanum onites* and *Origanum dubium*. If the label lists thyme (*Thymus vulgaris*) or marjoram (*Origanum majorana*) or a blend of oils, find another brand, because those herbs do not offer the same benefits.

Go organic. To limit your exposure to pesticides, look for oregano oil that has been steam distilled from organically grown plants.

Select pure oil. The only ingredient listed on the label should be the plant name with its botanical (Latin) name. If the oregano oil is diluted, the carrier oil should also be listed. There should be no additives.

Watch for false claims. Don't be fooled or confused by packaging that states "therapeutic" or "medicinal" grade. There are no such established standards for essential oils. These terms are primarily for marketing purposes.

Preparation

Essential oils can be used in a number of ways, from inhalation to massage to topical application on specific areas of the body. Like most pure essential oils, oregano essential oil is too potent to use full strength and, as mentioned on page 26, must be blended with a carrier oil, such as calendula, coconut, jojoba, olive, or sweet almond oil, before using on the skin. Author and botanist James Duke suggests diluting one or two drops of oregano essential oil in one tablespoon of vegetable oil; other experts suggest combining the oils at a ratio of 1:1 or 1:4. Clinical herbalist Michelle Lynde considers the ideal ratio to be one part essential oil to three parts carrier oil. Use caution the first time you try oregano essential oil by starting with a larger amount of carrier oil. When it comes to essential oils, more is *not* better. Use the smallest effective dose.

Before using oregano oil (or any essential oil) as a treatment, do a patch test on your skin to check for an allergic reaction or sensitivity. Mix a small amount of carrier oil, such as olive oil, with a few drops of the oregano oil at the ratio you plan to use for treatments. Using a cotton swab or dropper, put a small amount of the diluted oil on the inside of your elbow or wrist and cover with a bandage. If you feel any irritation, remove the bandage and wash the area with mild soap and water. If you've experienced no side effects after twenty-four hours, you can use the diluted oregano oil safely.

Note that oregano is considered a "hot" oil, which means it can burn or cause irritation even when diluted. So even if you have no reaction to it during the patch test, maintain caution when using the oil.

Methods and Treatments

The following two methods for using oregano oil––inhalation and topical application––can be helpful in treating a variety of conditions. You can easily try them at home.

Inhalation

Inhaling the scent of oregano oil is probably the easiest and safest way to relieve the stuffy nose and congestion that typically accompany a cold. It may also benefit asthma, bronchitis, flu, and sinus infections. For even more relief, use a combination of peppermint oil and oregano oil. You can use a diffuser or simply put a drop or two of the oil on a cotton ball or handkerchief. For a general feeling of well-being, try blending oregano's spicy, camphor-like aroma with earthy or citrusy scents, such as cedarwood, citronella, lavender, pine, or rosemary.

Topical Applications

The following remedies are rubbed into the skin, massaged over specific body parts, or applied to furniture or household surfaces:

Acne or rosacea. Combine equal amounts of oregano essential oil and coconut, jojoba, or olive oil and apply the mixture to the affected areas with a cotton swab once or twice a day until the condition clears up.

Arthritis. Apply a few drops of diluted oregano oil to the affected areas and gently massage into the skin to help reduce pain and inflammation. Alternatively, add 2 drops of the undiluted essential oil to warm bathwater.

Bug bites. Apply oregano essential oil diluted with olive oil to the bite. This may also help relieve poison ivy and other rashes.

Colds or sinus problems. Blend 2 drops of oregano essential oil with a carrier oil and gently massage the mixture into the bottoms of your feet. Alternatively, apply the mixture to your chest or back, or add it to warm bathwater.

Dandruff. Mix a few drops of oregano essential oil with your shampoo and work into your scalp. Avoid getting any of the oil in your eyes (it will sting). Do this for at least one week for maximum effect.

Digestion. Add 1 drop of oregano essential oil to a small amount of sesame oil or other carrier oil and rub on your abdomen to aid digestion.

Foot or nail fungus. Put several drops of oregano essential oil in a pan of water and soak your feet in it. You can also try blending 1 drop of oregano oil with a carrier oil and apply the mixture directly to your nails or feet. James Duke notes that using a mixture of antifungal essential oils may do an even better job. Try combining two parts of oregano essential oil with eight parts of tea tree oil and apply twice daily to the affected area. Alternatively, put the oil blend on a cotton ball and tape it right to the toenail.

Hand sanitizer. Combine 10 drops of oregano essential oil with 2 tablespoons of coconut oil. Rub the mixture into your hands, then let it soak in. This will also help nourish your skin and soften your hands.

Immune system boost. Rub oregano essential oil mixed with coconut oil on the bottoms of your feet.

Infections or allergies. To help ward off skin infections or allergies, blend 2 drops of oregano essential oil into a small amount of olive oil and apply topically to the affected areas. Alternatively, add 2 drops of oregano essential oil to your bath or mix the oil into your skin cream or lotion.

Insect repellent. Put a few drops of oregano essential oil on outdoor furniture (try a test spot first to make sure it doesn't stain), or apply diluted oregano essential oil on your skin before going outdoors.

Poison ivy and rashes. See "Bug bites," page 28.

Respiratory infection. A great way to fight a cold or respiratory infection is to put 1 drop of oregano essential oil in a pan of steaming water. Drape a towel loosely over your head and inhale the steam once a day until you feel better. If you're taking antibiotics, don't stop, and see your health care professional if symptoms don't improve.

Sore muscles. Create a mixture of half oregano essential oil and half olive oil and apply topically to the affected areas for relief. If you suffer from sore muscles, sports injuries, or backaches, this is definitely worth a try.

Stomach upset or gas. Add 2 or 3 drops of oregano essential oil to a warm compress and place on your abdomen. A compress is simply a clean cloth soaked in water that contains a few drops of essential oil.

Surface sanitizer. Put 10 drops of oregano essential oil in a 16-ounce spray bottle filled with water and spray over hard surfaces.

Oral Applications

The Alliance of International Aromatherapists advises against using essential oils internally. On its website (alliance-aromatherapists.org) it states: "AIA does not endorse internal therapeutic use (oral, vaginal, or rectal) of essential oils unless recommended by a health care practitioner trained at an appropriate clinical level. An appropriate level of training must include chemistry, anatomy, diagnostics, physiology, formulation guidelines, and safety issues regarding each specific internal route (oral, vaginal, or rectal)."

Noted aromatherapist Julia Lawless, author of *The Encyclopedia of Essential Oils*, also recommends using essential oils only externally, primarily because of the oils' high concentration and the potential to irritate or damage mucous membranes and the stomach lining. The oils will work just as well as topical applications since they are absorbed into the skin and are easily transported throughout the body.

If you plan to use an oral treatment, including those below, do so only under the guidance of a licensed, experienced practitioner. (While these are oral applications, they do not involve swallowing the oil.)

Bad breath or plaque. Add 1 drop of oregano oil to your toothpaste.

Parasites or infections. Dilute oregano essential oil with a carrier oil and put 1 drop under your tongue. Hold it there for a few minutes and then rinse it out. Repeat four times a day.

Sore throat. Mix 1 or 2 drops of oregano essential oil with a small amount of water and gargle. Alternatively, simply sip a cup of tea made with fresh or dried oregano leaves (see page 36).

Safety Precautions

Follow these additional guidelines when using and storing oregano essential oil:

- Always store oregano essential oil in a cool place in dark bottles and away from direct sunlight (to protect from photo oxidation), allowing as little contact with air as possible. The shelf life of most essential oils is about two years.

- Keep oregano essential oil (and all essential oils, which are flammable) away from heat sources and out of reach of children.

- Allergic reactions to oregano essential oil, such as skin rashes or anaphylaxis, are rare.

- Because oregano essential oil in its pure form is so strong, it should only be used when diluted. Undiluted, it can be irritating to the skin and mucous membranes.

- Don't use diluted oregano essential oil on broken skin, cuts, scrapes, or sensitive skin, as it can cause irritation.

- Do not exceed recommended dosages, as doing so can cause stomach upset, rashes, or skin irritation. Large doses can be toxic.

- Oregano essential oil is not intended for long-term use, so use it for just a week or two and then take a break. Extended exposure may cause irritation.

- Avoid contact with eyes, mouth, nasal passages, and genital areas.

- People who take lithium or have gallbladder, kidney, or liver disease should avoid oregano essential oil. Some sources suggest that people with high blood pressure or a heart condition should avoid using the oil as well. Individuals allergic to basil, lavender, hyssop, marjoram, and mint should also not use it.

- Oregano essential oil may inhibit the absorption of iron, so people prone to anemia should not use it often.

- Oregano essential oil is not advised for use with infants, children younger than two years of age, and pregnant or nursing women.

Conclusion

Scientific research as of this writing has not proven that oregano essential oil can effectively treat such conditions as rheumatoid arthritis, urinary tract infections, herpes simplex, or cancer, although consumers are bound to find such claims online and in other media. While the findings from several studies show promise for oregano's antibacterial, antifungal, anti-inflammatory, antioxidant, antiparasitic, and antiviral benefits, sufficient human testing is lacking. "The therapeutic potential of essential oils has yet to be realized," writes Julia Lawless. So for now it's up to consumers to educate themselves by talking to herbalists and health care providers, reading about other consumers' experiences and how oil of oregano is used around the world, and using the herb and its essential oil wisely, as you would any other remedy.

Using the Oregano Plant

Using fresh or dried oregano leaves when you simmer a sauce, toss a salad, brew a tea, or make an infusion can deliver some of the same nutritional and healing benefits of the plant without the potential toxicity of the essential oil. The trade-off, however, is that there is also less potency. When you grow your own oregano, you not only save money but also control the herb's quality and flavor by avoiding pesticides and having access to the freshest herb possible. Below are guidelines for how to grow and store the most flavorful oregano.

Growing Oregano

Oregano plants can be started from seeds or cuttings six to ten weeks before the last spring frost, according to the *Old Farmer's Almanac*. Oregano, like many herbs, loves the sun, and strong sunlight will help give the plant a strong flavor.

Make sure to plant oregano in well-drained soil; if your soil retains too much moisture, you may want to grow the herb in a container or a raised vegetable garden. Because oregano's water needs are moderate, wait until the soil seems dry to the touch and then water thoroughly. Too much moisture may result in root rot.

After the oregano has grown to about four inches, trim it slightly to help it branch out and become bushier. Then trim it every so often to avoid the plant from getting leggy. If you want to share cuttings with friends, perennial oregano can be divided in early spring.

Oregano leaves are at their most flavorful right before the plant's flowers bloom. Pick in the morning after the dew has dried but before the hot afternoon sun wilts the plants. Choose firm stems and leaves that are vibrant green without yellowing or dark spots. To use the fresh leaves in cooking, cut them from their stems, wash the leaves, and pat them dry. Then roll them between your hands to crush and release their natural oils.

Wrapped in a damp paper towel and stored in a plastic bag, fresh oregano will keep in the refrigerator for up to three days. If you can't use up your fresh harvest fast enough, consider freezing or drying it (see the sections that follow) for future use.

Freezing Oregano

Oregano leaves freeze well. Here are two easy freezing methods:

Method 1: Wash, drain, and pat dry the leaves, then spread them on a baking sheet and put in the freezer. Once the leaves are frozen, transfer them to ziplock bags or air-tight containers. Make sure to label the bag or container with the name of the herb and the date. If you chop the oregano for recipes before freezing it, also include the quantity on the label.

Method 2: Another way to freeze chopped fresh oregano is in an ice-cube tray. Once you've chopped the leaves, measure out 1 tablespoon into each compartment, add water, and freeze. When you need 1 tablespoon of oregano for cooking, simply pop out a cube and thaw it.

Drying Oregano

Because of oregano's intense flavor, some cooks maintain that dried oregano is preferable to fresh in cooking. That's because drying the herb can help diminish its bitterness while retaining its potent taste. If you want to dry at least part of your harvest, doing it naturally will preserve the most flavor and oil content. However, drying oregano in the oven or microwave, or in the sun, will deplete both.

First snip several healthy stems and rinse them lightly in water. Shake off the excess moisture and let the stems dry thoroughly to avoid mold. Then bundle four to six branches together with string or a rubber band and hang the stems upside down away from direct sunlight in a warm, dry, well-ventilated area. This method can become messy as the leaves dry, so you may want to place the bundles in paper bags to catch any debris. Cut slits or punch holes in the bags to allow the air to circulate. Drying should take between one and two weeks. After the oregano has dried, remove any flowers, then strip the stems of the leaves by running your fingers down the branch. For the fullest flavor, the dried leaves should be stored whole in an airtight glass jar or similar container and crushed just before adding to a dish. Stored in a dark place, such as a pantry or cupboard, the dried leaves should keep for about six months. Make sure to label the jar with the name of the herb and the date.

If the above method is too time consuming, you can simply spread the leaves on a baking sheet or pan and let them air-dry, uncovered. In general, one-quarter teaspoon of powdered oregano is equal to one teaspoon of crushed dried oregano or one tablespoon of chopped fresh oregano. A little oregano goes a long way.

Buying Fresh Oregano

No time to grow your own oregano? No problem! Produce departments at local grocery stores are most likely to carry either Mediterranean or Mexican oregano. Their flavors are similar, but the Mexican variety (*Lippia graveolens*) is more pungent and less sweet than the Mediterranean kind, which may be sold as "Greek oregano" or "Turkish oregano." The Mexican variety partners well with cumin and chili powder, while the European variety complements mildly flavored dishes, such as grains and vegetables.

Recipes

Oregano Tea

Makes 1 cup

Sip this strong tea to soothe a sore throat or open stuffy sinuses. Gargling with the unsweetened tea also may help relieve mouth irritations. In some parts of the world, oregano tea is used to treat insomnia and anxiety. Chopping or crushing the leaves helps release their beneficial compounds into the water. To temper oregano's slightly bitter flavor, add sugar or other sweetener to taste. Three cups a day is a common recommendation, since tea is not as potent as other forms of herbal remedies. Serve the tea hot, iced, or at room temperature.

> 1 cup boiling water
> 1 tablespoon chopped fresh oregano leaves, or 1 teaspoon dried
>   oregano leaves
> Sugar, agave nectar, stevia, or other sweetener (optional)

Pour the water into a teacup. Add the oregano and let steep for 10 minutes. Strain. Sweeten to taste if desired.

Tip: Renowned herbalist, teacher, and author Rosemary Gladstar writes that tea is her favorite way to use herbs medicinally, even though tea is not as potent as other herbal remedies. She recommends making 1 quart of tea at a time instead of 1 cup and storing it in the refrigerator, where it will keep for 3 to 4 days.

Lemony Garlic Salad Dressing

Makes about ¾ cup

This light dressing adds pizzazz to a Greek salad or any combination of fresh greens and veggies.

½ cup olive oil

¼ cup freshly squeezed lemon juice

1 clove garlic, minced

½ teaspoon dried oregano

Sea salt

Freshly ground black pepper

Put the oil, lemon juice, garlic, and oregano in a small bowl and whisk until emulsified. Season with salt and pepper taste. Transfer to a small jar, seal tightly, and store in the refrigerator. Shake well before using.

Variation: For extra zip, add Dijon mustard to taste.

Oregano Pesto

Makes 1 cup

Making pesto is a flavorful way to use the bounty of oregano from your garden. Enjoy the pesto on pasta, in sandwiches and omelets, mixed with roasted vegetables, or as an appetizer spread on crackers or baguette slices. It freezes well too.

2 cups stemmed fresh oregano leaves, firmly packed

½ cup pine nuts, lightly toasted

3 cloves garlic

½ cup olive oil

Sea salt

Freshly ground pepper

Put the oregano, pine nuts, and garlic in a food processor and pulse until coarsely ground, about 30 seconds. With the processor running, slowly drizzle in the oil. Season with salt and pepper to taste and pulse until evenly distributed.

Variation: Traditional pesto uses fresh basil and Parmesan cheese. Feel free to use a mixture of oregano and basil in this recipe. To add a cheesy flavor, blend in 3 tablespoons of nutritional yeast or vegan Parmesan cheese.

Herbes de Provence

Makes 9 tablespoons

There are many versions of this classic seasoning blend, which is based on herbs that thrive in the south of France. Most mixtures include coarsely crumbled dried thyme and savory. Try this classic blend sprinkled over salads, stirred into soups or stews, or mixed with olive oil as a dipping sauce for crusty bread. Once you try the recipe as written, experiment with your own herbal combinations, using additions such as dried basil, parsley, sage, tarragon, or lavender flowers, or even fennel seeds and orange zest.

3 tablespoons dried thyme

2 tablespoons dried oregano

2 tablespoons dried savory

1 tablespoon dried marjoram

1 tablespoon dried rosemary

Crumble the herbs into a small jar and shake until well combined. Seal tightly and store at room temperature. For a finer texture, pulse briefly in a food processor or crush with a mortar and pestle.

Summer Garden Ratatouille

Makes 4 servings

Easy and flavorful, this vegetable stew combines homegrown favorites, such as zucchini, tomatoes, and bell pepper. Serve it on its own or over couscous or rice.

> 2 tablespoons olive oil
>
> 1 large red onion, diced
>
> 2 cloves garlic, minced
>
> 1 medium eggplant, peeled and cubed
>
> ½ cup vegetable broth
>
> 2 large, ripe tomatoes, chopped
>
> 2 small zucchini, cubed
>
> 2 small yellow squash, cubed
>
> 1 red bell pepper, chopped
>
> 1 tablespoon finely chopped fresh oregano leaves
>
> Sea salt
>
> Freshly ground black pepper
>
> ¼ cup pitted oil-cured olives, chopped

Put the oil in a large skillet over medium heat. When hot, add the onion and garlic and cook, stirring frequently, until the onion has softened slightly, about 3 minutes. Add the eggplant and broth and cook, stirring occasionally, until the eggplant is tender, about 10 minutes. Add the tomatoes, zucchini, yellow squash, and bell pepper and cook, stirring occasionally, until the zucchini and yellow squash are tender but firm, 9 to 10 minutes. Stir in the oregano and cook for 1 minute longer. Season with salt and pepper to taste. Garnish with the olives.

Tip: In a hurry? Instead of fresh tomatoes, substitute one 14-ounce can of diced tomatoes with juice. Instead of fresh oregano, use 1½ teaspoons of dried oregano and add it with the tomatoes.

OREGANO OIL INFUSIONS **41**

Oregano Oil Infusions

Unlike essential oils that are produced by a steam-distillation process, infusions (also called herb-infused oils) are similar to making tea but the leaves are steeped for a longer period of time. Making infused oils is easy to do at home. There are a handful of variations on the basic method—cold infusion; solar infusion; and heat infusion, using the stovetop or oven or a double boiler—and recipes using these methods are readily available on the web.

Some sites invite visitors to "make your own oil of oregano," but the method is actually for an oil infusion, not an essential oil. Some at-home methods use fresh oregano, but others call for the dried herb. Using the dried form will prevent the growth of mold or bacteria and give the infusion a longer shelf life.

Infusions Using Dried Oregano Leaves

To make an oil-based infusion with dried oregano leaves, you'll need the dried herb; olive, almond, or melted coconut oil; and a clean, sanitized glass jar. Fill the jar halfway with dried oregano leaves and add enough oil to cover the oregano completely. Stir to remove any air bubbles. Gently turn or shake the jar to make sure all the leaves are covered with the oil. Put the jar in a warm place out of direct sunlight. If the only warm spot is in the sun, put the jar in a paper bag to protect the leaves from the sun's rays. Let the oil steep for 4 to 6 weeks. Turn or shake the jar every few days. After 5 weeks, strain the oil through cheesecloth into another clean, sanitized glass jar and seal tightly. Store the infused oil in a cool, dry place. It should keep for about 1 year.

Infusions Using Fresh Oregano Leaves

To make an oil-based infusion using fresh oregano leaves, first make sure the herb is completely dry. Any moisture could cause the oil to become moldy or rancid. Fill a clean, sanitized glass jar about halfway with the fresh oregano leaves and cover with olive, almond, or melted coconut oil. Stir gently to remove any air bubbles. Fill a small saucepan two-thirds full with water and heat to a rolling boil. Remove from the heat. Set the jar in the water and let stand for 5 to 10 minutes to allow the oregano to release its natural oils. Remove the jar from the water bath, pat dry, and put it in a warm spot. Turn or shake the jar every few days. After 1 to 2 weeks, strain the oil through cheesecloth into a clean, sanitized glass jar. Seal tightly. Store the infused oil in a cool, dry place. It should keep for about 1 year.

Alternative Infusion Methods

The following methods can be used for either fresh or dried oregano leaves:

Method 1: Preheat the oven to 250 degrees F, then turn it off. Put fresh or dried oregano leaves in a clean baking pan and cover with olive, almond, or melted coconut oil. Put the uncovered pan in the oven for 24 hours. Strain the oil through cheesecloth into a clean, sanitized glass jar.

Method 2: Fill a clean, sanitized glass jar about halfway with the fresh oregano leaves and cover with olive, almond, or melted coconut oil. Stir gently to remove any air bubbles. Heat a slow cooker, dehydrator, or yogurt maker on the warm setting (100 to 120 degrees F). Put the jar with the herb and oil in the slow cooker, dehydrator, or yogurt maker for 8 to 12 hours, occasionally turning or shaking the jar. Let cool. Strain the oil through cheesecloth into a clean, sanitized glass jar.

Suggested Uses

Oregano oil infusions are ideal to use in homemade lotions, salves, and rubs. The infused oil can also be applied directly as a remedy for arthritis, carpal tunnel syndrome, cold sores, sore muscles, insect bites and stings, nail fungus, and toothaches. Even though an infusion is not as potent as an essential oil, you should still do a skin test before using the infusion as a topical treatment or adding it to homemade skin care products.

Homemade Oregano Salve

Makes 1¼ cups

4 to 6 ounces oregano oil infusion

1 cup grated or shaved beeswax

Pour the infused oil into the top portion of a double boiler or into a glass container, such as a measuring cup, and set it in a saucepan of water. Warm the oil over low heat and gradually add the beeswax, stirring until melted. Pour into clean, dry tins or glass jars and store in a cool, dark place. The salve will keep for about 1 year.

Tip: Before pouring into containers, test the texture of the salve by putting 1 teaspoon of the mixture in the refrigerator for 1 minute. If the salve comes out too soft, add more beeswax. If it's too hard, add more oil for a creamier consistency.

Variation: To enhance the salve's medicinal benefits, stir in 10 drops of oregano essential oil just before pouring the mixture into containers.

References

Ahuja, Akshay. 2014. "Living Medicine: Stephen Harrod Buhner on Plant Intelligence, Natural Healing, and the Trouble with Pharmaceuticals." *The Sun*, December.

Basilico, M. Z., and J. C. Basilico. 1999. "Inhibitory Effects of Some Spice Essential Oils on *Aspergillus ochraceus* NRRL 3174 Growth and Ochratoxin A Production." *Letters in Applied Microbiology* 4:238-41. http://goo.gl/DDkU1M.

Bliss, Rosalie Marion. 2002. "Herbs Can Spice Up Your Antioxidant Protection." US Department of Agriculture Agricultural Research Service. Last modified March 5. http://goo.gl/uhyXBt.

Boon, Heather, and Michael Smith. 2009. *55 Most Common Medicinal Herbs*, 2nd ed. Toronto: Robert Rose, Inc.

Bower, A. M., L. M. Real Hernandez, M. A. Berhow, and E. Gonzalez de Mejia. 2014. "Bioactive Compounds from Culinary Herbs Inhibit a Molecular Target for Type 2 Diabetes Management, Dipeptidyl Peptidase IV." *Journal of Agricultural and Food Chemistry* 62 (26):6147–58.

Braga, P. C., M. Dal Sasso, M. Culici, T. Bianchi, L. Bordoni, and L. Marabini. 2006. "Anti-inflammatory Activity of Thymol: Inhibitory Effect on the Release of Human Neutrophil Elastase." *Pharmacology* 77 (3):130–6.

Centers for Disease Control and Prevention. 2013. "National Health Interview Survey 2012." http://goo.gl/ICmBlj.

Cleff, M. B., A. R. Meinerz, M. Xavier, L. F. Schuch, M. C. Araújo Meireles, M. R. Alves Rodrigues, and J. R. Braga de Mello. 2010. "*In Vitro* Activity of *Origanum vulgare* Essential Oil against *Candida* Species." *Brazilian Journal of Microbiology* 41 (1): 116–23. http://goo.gl/R997K6.

Coles, Terri. 2013. "Oil of Oregano Benefits: 11 Things to Know About Oregano Oil." Huffington Post Canada. Last modified January 7, 2016. http://goo.gl/Y6dbOC.

Duke, James. 1997. *The Green Pharmacy*. Emmaus, PA: Rodale Press.

El Babili, F., J. Bouajila, J. P. Souchard, C. Bertrand, F. Bellvert, I. Fouraste, C. Moulis, and A. Valentin. 2011. "Oregano: Chemical Analysis and Evaluation of Its Antimalarial, Antioxidant, and Cytotoxic Activities." *Journal of Food Science* 76 (April):C512–8.

Force, M., W. S. Sparks, and R. A. Ronzio. 2000. "Inhibition of Enteric Parasites by Emulsified Oil of Oregano *in Vivo*." *Phytotherapy Research* 14 (May):213–214.

Foster, Karen. 2013. "Oregano: One of the Most Beneficial Spices for Our Health with Four Times the Antioxidant Potency of Blueberries." PreventDisease.com. October 7. http://goo.gl/k064t0.

Fritz, Heidi. 2015. "Oil of Oregano: Properties and Uses." *Naturopathic Currents*. March 9. http://goo.gl/LG3rNO.

Georgetown University Medical Center. 2001. "Oregano Oil May Protect Against Drug-Resistant Bacteria, Georgetown Researcher Finds." *Science Daily*. October 11. http://goo.gl/0HGtFJ.

Gilling, D. H., M. Kitajima, J. R. Torrey, and K. R. Bright. 2014. "Antiviral Efficacy and Mechanisms of Action of Oregano Essential Oil and Its Primary Component Carvacrol against Murine Norovirus." *Journal of Applied Microbiology* 116 (May):1149–1163.

Gladstar, Rosemary. 2012. "How to Make Herbal Teas, Herbal Infusions, and Herbal Tinctures." *Mother Earth News*, February 9. http://goo.gl/fkPTQf.

Greenspan, H. C., and Aruoma OI, 1994. "Oxidative Stress and Apoptosis in HIV Infection: A Role for Plant-Derived Metabolites with Synergistic Antioxidant Activity. *Immunology Today* 15(5):209–13. http://goo.gl/rJBXDh.

Harpaz, S., L. Glatman, V. Drabkin, and A. Gelman. 2003. "Effects of Herbal Essential Oils Used to Extend the Shelf Life of Freshwater-Reared Asian Sea Bass Fish (Lates calcarifer)." *Journal of Food Protection* 66 (3):410–17. http://goo.gl/4mwQcF.

Herb Society of America. 2005. *Oregano and Marjoram: An Herb Society of America Guide to the Genus Origanum*. herbsociety.org.

Herbal Academy of New England. herbalacademyofne.com.

Hyldgaard, M., T. Mygind, and R. L. Meyer. 2012. "Essential Oils in Food Preservation: Mode of Action, Synergies, and Interactions with Food Matrix Components." *Frontiers in Microbiology* 3:12.

Kulisic, T., A. Radonic, V. Katalinic, and M. Milos. 2004. "Use of Different Methods for Testing Antioxidative Activity of Oregano Essential Oil." *Food Chemistry* 85 (40):633–640. https://goo.gl/7blXsE.

Kulisic, T., A. Krisko, V. Dragovic-Uzelac, M. Milos, and G. Pifat. 2007. "The Effects of Essential Oils and Aqueous Tea Infusions of Oregano (*Origanum vulgare* L. spp. *hirtum*), Thyme (*Thymus vulgaris* L.), and Wild Thyme (*Thymus serpyllum* L.) on the Copper-Induced Oxidation of Human Low-Density Lipoproteins." *International Journal of Food Sciences and Nutrition* 58 (2):87–93. http://goo.gl/cptd6o.

Lawless, Julia. 2013. *The Encyclopedia of Essential Oils*. San Francisco: Conari Press.

Martin-Sanchez, A. M., C. Chaves-Lopez, E. Sendra, E. Savas, J. Fenandez-Lopez, and J. A. Perez-Alvarez. 2011. "Lipolysis, Proteolysis, and Sensory Characteristics of a Spanish Fermented Dry-Cured Meat Product (Salchichón) with Oregano Essential Oil Used as Surface Mold Inhibitor." *Meat Science* 89 (1):35–44.

Martyris, Nina. 2015. "GIs Helped Bring Freedom to Europe and a Taste for Oregano to America." National Public Radio. May 15. http://goo.gl/zgKZpZ.

Mercola, Joseph. 2014. "What Are the Health Benefits of Oregano?" Mercola.com. February 1. http://goo.gl/SXI7I9.

Monaco, Lisa, and Dr. John P. Holdren. 2014. "New Executive Actions to Combat Anti-biotic Resistance and Protect Public Health." The White House. September 14. https://goo.gl/o7T3Zt.

National Institutes of Health. "Complementary and Alternative Medicine." https://goo.gl/lKmCWq.

National Institutes of Health. 2014. "Stop the Spread of Superbugs." February. https://goo.gl/MLPS8p.

Nolte, Kurt. "Oregano." University of Arizona, Yuma County Cooperative Extension. http://goo.gl/u27R9v.

Nurmi, A., T. Nurmi, J. Mursu, R. Hiltunen, and S. Voutilainen. 2006. "Ingestion of Oregano Extract Increases Excretion of Urinary Phenolic Metabolites in Humans." *Journal of Agricultural and Food Chemistry* 54 (18):6916–23.

Old Farmer's Almanac. "Oregano." almanac.com.

Osakabe, N., H. Takano, C. Sanbongi, A. Yasuda, R. Yanagisawa, K. Inoue, and T. Yoshikawa. 2004. "Anti-Inflammatory and Anti-Allergic Effect of Rosmarinic Acid (RA); Inhibition of Seasonal Allergic Rhinoconjunctivitis (SAR) and Its Mechanism." *Biofactors* 21 (1–4):127–131.

Paddock, Catharine. 2008. "Himalayan Oregano Effective against MRSA." *Medical News Today*, November 24. http://goo.gl/2Dms4p.

Prior, Ronald. 2012. "Antioxidant Food Databases? Valuable or Not?" (response to the USDA ORAC statement), http://goo.gl/zUT6jp.

Reinagel, Monica. 2013. "What Are ORAC Values?" *Scientific American*, August 14. http://goo.gl/fzjMfp.

Rodriguez, Tori. 2015. "Essential Oils Might Be the New Antibiotics." *The Atlantic*, January 15. http://goo.gl/WaBNAI.

Sahelian, Ray, MD. 2014. "ORAC Value of Foods, Acai, Mangosteen, and Others." February 12. http://goo.gl/fKuuxZ.

Singletary, Keith. 2010. "MSI Funded Paper: Potential Health Benefits of Oregano." McCormick Science Institute. August. http://goo.gl/Zijbnm.

Soo Xi Yap, P., B. C. Yiap, H. C. Ping, and S. H. Lim. 2014. "Essential Oils, A New Horizon in Combating Bacterial Antibiotic Resistance." *Open Microbiology Journal* 8:6–14.

Strom, Stephanie. 2012. "In Hopes of Healthier Chickens, Farms Turn to Oregano." *New York Times*, December 25. http://goo.gl/vngCt6.

The Dr. Oz Show. 2014. "Oil of Oregano Guide." January 16. http://goo.gl/30uJmZ.

Tillotson, Alan Keith. 2001. *The One Earth Herbal Sourcebook.* New York: Kensington Publishing Corp.

University of Maryland Medical Center. "Herbal Medicine: Overview." Last reviewed November 6, 2015. http://goo.gl/MWzykO.

World Health Net. 2009. "Oregano Helps Stop Inflammation and Bone Degeneration." May 28. http://goo.gl/XV7edr.

Xu, J., F. Zhou, B. P. Ji, R. S. Pei, and N. Xu. 2008. "The Antibacterial Mechanism of Carvacrol and Thymol against *Escherichia coli.*" *Letters in Applied Microbiology* 47 (3):174–9.

About the Author

Barbara Schuetz is a Wisconsin-based writer and editor who has covered a variety of food, health, and lifestyle topics for newspapers and magazines, including *Taste of Home.*

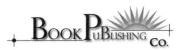

Book Publishing Co.
books that educate, inspire, and empower

All titles in the **Live Healthy Now** series are only **$5.95**!

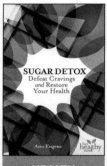 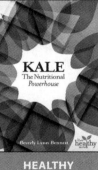 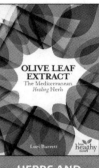 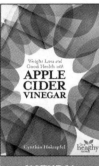

HEALTH ISSUES	HEALTHY FOODS	HERBS AND SUPPLEMENTS	NATURAL SOLUTIONS
SUGAR DETOX Defeat Cravings and Restore Your Health	**KALE** The Nutritional Powerhouse	**OLIVE LEAF EXTRACT** The Mediterranean Healing Herb	Weight Loss and Good Health with **APPLE CIDER VINEGAR**
GLUTEN-FREE Success Strategies	Enhance Your Health with **FERMENTED FOODS**	**AROMATHERAPY** Essential Oils for Healing	Healthy and Beautiful with **COCONUT OIL**
A Holistic Approach to **ADHD**	**GREEN SMOOTHIES:** The Easy Way to Get Your Greens	The Pure Power of **MACA**	The Weekend **DETOX**
Understanding **GOUT**	**PALEO** Smoothies		Improve Digestion with **FOOD COMBINING**
WHEAT BELLY– Is Modern Wheat Causing Modern Ills?	Refreshing Fruit and Vegetable **SMOOTHIES**		The Healing Power of **TURMERIC**
The **ACID-ALKALINE** Diet			

Interested in other health topics or healthy cookbooks? See our complete line of titles at **BookPubCo.com** or order directly from:
Book Publishing Company • P.O. Box 99 • Summertown, TN 38483 • 1-888-260-8458